Dr. High Yield's Psychiatry Notes
(for the Step 2 CK & Shelf Exams)

Steven K. M. Vuu, M.D.

DEDICATION

to all sentient beings

CONTENTS

ACKNOWLEDGMENTS

To my family (Mom, Dad, Andrew), teachers, colleagues, and all those who have helped me along the way, I wouldn't be where I am today without you. Thank you.

DR. HIGH YIELD'S PSYCHIATRY NOTES

Introduction:

These are my never before seen notes I used to prepare for my Step 2 CK and shelf board examinations. It is basically a conglomeration of all the books I read and the practice questions I did during 3rd year medical school. The notes are written in a short form, casual manner, deliberately. I used it as a way to cement knowledge and maximize repetitions before the exam. Before you read this, remember that this is not meant to be a primary study resource. These notes are meant to supplement your baseline studies, you should already have an understanding of the basics. This is for a quick review of potent things you might have overlooked or forgotten. These bullet points are meant to be quickly read through. They will help you zone in on key details and equip you with knowledge to help answer a question you may encounter. It is in numbered form on purpose. This helps you keep focus and know how far along you are without losing your place in the list. It is best used as a last minute read the last few days prior to the exam where you don't have enough time to read a textbook or do more practice questions. If you are having trouble understanding, then go back to the source textbook or question bank and fill in the details as you wish. Best of luck on your exam. Enjoy!

Abbreviations:

1. tx/rx = treat
2. sx = symptoms
3. dx = diagnosis
4. ddx = differential diagnosis
5. dz = disease
6. a/w = associated with
7. OHTN = orthostatic hypotension
8. AE = adverse effect
9. SE = side effect
10. HAM block = antihistamine, alpha blockade, antimuscarinic
11. benzo = benzodiazepine
12. CBT = cognitive behavioral therapy
13. NCD = neurocognitive disorder
14. MDD = major depressive disorder
15. ECT = electroconvulsive therapy
16. EPS = extrapyramidal symptoms
17. 2/2 = secondary to
18. a/w = associated with
19. CI = contraindication
20. w/u = work up
21. f/u = follow up
22. w/ = with
23. LN = lymph node
24. u/s or us = ultrasound
25. abx = antibiotics

****

Things to Keep in Mind When Doing Questions:

1. **rule out** the other answers
2. if u know one of them to be true and are unsure then **pick the one u know to be true**
3. if u dont know **pick the more common things**
4. **keep it simple**
5. if u dont know **move on quick** and take the L on that question and move on to save time and get other ones right
6. **age** is important
7. put the **whole picture** together
8. when it comes down to 2 answers, try to reject one of them

PSYCHIATRIC EMERGENCY TREATMENTS

1. Neuroleptic malignant syndrome = discontinue + dantrolene
2. Serotonin syndrome = discontinue + benzos or cyproheptadine
3. Tyramine crisis = nitroprusside or phentolamine
4. acute dystonia = benztropine or benadryl
5. lithium toxicity = hydrate aggressively or hemodialysis
6. TCA toxicity = sodium bicarb (unblocks the sodium channels in the heart)
7. cocaine overdose = benzo
8. alcohol withdrawal = benzo
9. Delirium tremens = benzos
10. PCP overdose = benzo
11. benzo overdose = flumazenil
12. benzo withdrawal = benzo taper
13. opioid overdose = naloxone
14. opioid withdrawal = clonidine BP support

PSYCHOTIC DISORDERS

1. visual/tactile hallucinations = drug intoxication, drug/alcohol withdrawal, delirium
2. olfactory hallucination = epilepsy
3. important workup for possible schizophrenia = thyroid, syphilis, b12, polypharmacy, electrolytes
4. echolalia = repeats words or phrases
5. echopraxia = mimics behavior (practices behavior)
6. 5 A's of negative symptoms of schizophrenia = anhedonia = no interest, affect (loss of) = no emotion, avolition = no motivation, alogia = no speech, no attention; schizophrenia patients may present with negative symptoms
7. men get schizophrenia early 20s
8. females get schizophrenia late 20s
9. men have more negative symptoms
10. highly genetic component to schizophrenia (twins 50% chance the other will have it)
11. lifetime prevalence of schizophrenia is 0.3-0.7%
12. antipsychotics block dopamine -> increase prolactin -> gynecomastia (tuberoinfundibular) especially risperidone
13. antipsychotics block substantia nigra -> parkinson like symptoms
14. good prognosis of schizophrenia = late onset, female, acute onset
15. poor prognosis of schizophrenia = early onset, male, family history, slow onset
16. 4 pathways = mesolimbic (positive sx), mesocortical (neg sx), tuberoinfundibular (hyperprolactinemia, gynecomastia), substantia nigra (parkinsonism)
17. brain imaging of schizophrenia = enlarged ventricles + diffuse cortical atrophy + reduced brain volume

18. second gen atypical neuroleptics = all end in -apine or -done
    1. lower risk of EPS but increased for metabolic syndrome
    2. should check BMI, BP, glucose, lipids
    3. risperidone famous for prolactinemia, olanzapine famous for metabolic syndrome
19. EPS antidotes
    1. dystonia = benzo or benadryl
    2. akathisia = beta blocker or benzo
    3. parkinsonism = benztropine
    4. tardive dyskinesia = valbenazine OR stop the medication, switch to clozapine
20. NMS = fever, rigidity, elevated WBC, metabolic acidosis, elevated creatine phosphokinase; antidote = stop med first, then dantrolene
21. thioRidazine AE = Retinal pigmentation
22. Chlorpromazine AE = Corneal deposits
23. schizoaffective = schizophrenia + depression OR schizophrenia + mania
    1. need to have schizophrenia for 2 weeks without mood disorder symptoms to rule out mood disorder with psychotic features (ensures that you are baseline psychotic)
    2. rx = second gen antipsychotic, mood stabilizers
24. brief psychotic disorder = <1 mo = reaction to extreme stress such as bereavement, sexual assault etc
    1. most recover completely
    2. give antipsychotics, benzos for agitation
25. schizophreniform = 1 to 6 month, schizophrenia = 6 month+; hallucinations, delusions, disorganized speech, negative symptoms
26. delusional disorder
    1. need at least 1 month of delusions only

2. functioning NORMALLY in society/occupation (MUST KNOW)
3. erotomanic type = believes someone is in love with them
4. rx = antipsychotics even tho poor evidence

27. best to worst prognosis: mood disorder with psychotic features > schizoaffective > schizophreniform > schizophrenia (moody stuff is better than psychotic stuff)

MOOD DISORDERS

1. mood episode = major depressive episode, mania, hypomania
2. mood disorder = major depressive disorder, bipolar disorder, persistent depressive disorder, cyclothymic
3. major depressive episode = at least 5 symptoms for 2 weeks+ of msigecaps
   1. m = decreased mood
   2. s = sleep changes
   3. i = loss of interest
   4. g = guilt
   5. e = loss of energy
   6. c = loss of concentration
   7. a = change in appetite
   8. p = psychomotor changes = sluggish
   9. s = suicidality
4. bipolar DIGFAST = distracted, insomnia, grandiose, flight of ideas, activity, speech, thoughtless
5. mania = at least 3 of DIGFAST for 1 week with impairment/hospitalization
6. hypomanic = at least 3 of DIGFAST for 4 days in a row without social/occupational impairment
7. must rule out medical causes first
   1. medical causes of depression = CVD, endocrinopathies, parkinsons, carcinoid, cancers, lupus
   2. medical causes of mania = thyroid, multiple sclerosis, cancer, HIV
   3. medication causes of depression = antihypertensives, corticosteroids, levodopa
   4. medication causes of bipolar = corticosteroids, levodopa, bronchodilators
8. major depressive disorder = at least one major depressive

episode + no history of bipolar

    1. onset peak in 20s

    2. 2x more common in women

    3. increases mortality in diabetes, stroke, cvd

    4. harder to go to sleep, wake up early, light sleeper, longer REM duration

    5. decreased CSF 5HIAA levels

    6. hyperactive cortisol axis

    7. abnormal thyroid axis

    8. 10% eventually commit suicide

    9. First thing about depressed pt is assess for risk of suicide to determine if u need to admit them

9. hamilton depression rating scale = measures severity of depression

10. PHQ9 = depression screening test

11. SSRI main SE = SHIGA = sexual, HA, insomnia, GI disturbance, appetite

12. mirtazapine = alpha 2 antagonist and 5ht2,3 antagonist (shunt 5ht to 5ht1) = makes u hungry and sleepy

13. TCA SE = HAM block + TRI Cs = antihistamine, alpha blocking, antimuscarinic, cardiac (long qt + arrhythmias), convulsions, coma

    1. HAM = histamine, alpha1, muscarinic

14. MAOIs = used for refractory depression = phenelzine

    1. wine, beer, aged cheese, smoked meat = tyramine; can lead to tyramine crisis

    2. risk of serotonin syndrome when mixed with SSRI

    3. most common side effect = ORTHOSTATIC HYPOTENSION

15. antidepressants take 4-6 weeks to fully work

    1. if working but side effects = switch SSRI

    2. if not working at all = switch drug classes

16. atypical depression first line = SSRI
    1. mood reactivity
    2. leaden paralysis
    3. hypersomnia
    4. hyperphagia
    5. sensitive to rejection
17. Electroconvulsive Therapy (ECT) = for emergencies = if need rapid changes like suicide risk or refusal to eat or drink = most efficacy form of tx for depression
    1. retrograde and anterograde amnesia resolves within 6 months
18. Catatonia = purposeless motor activity, immobility, bizarre postures like waxy flexibility or statue like, echolalia; rx = LORAZEPAM
19. Seasonal Affective Disorder triad = in cold dark northern locations, irritable, carb craving, hypersomnia, rx = light therapy
20. main thing that distinguishes peripartum blues vs peripartum depression = inability to enjoy their child is a sign of peripartum depression
21. bereavement = simple grief, does not include psychotic sx, disorganization, or suicidality, main factor vs depression = moments of improved mood, no feelings of worthlessness
    1. Grief u are still functioning and have good and bad days vs mdd
22. major depression with psychotic features rx = antidepressant + antipsychotic
23. mania with psychotic features rx = mood stabilizer + antipsychotic
24. bipolar 1 can have psychotic features, therefore if someone is psychotic always include bipolar as a ddx
25. rapid cycling = 4 or more mood episodes in 1 year rx = valproate = mood stabilizer

26. bipolar 1 = high income countries, before age 30, HIGHEST GENETIC LINK OF ALL PSYCHIATRIC DISORDERS, highly recurrent, poorer prognosis than MDD
27. lithium = ONLY MOOD STABILIZER THAT REDUCES SUICIDE RISK, low therapeutic index dangerous; overdose tx = dialysis
28. top 2 SE of lithium = weight gain, tremor and LMNOP mnemonic = lithium, movement disorder, nephrogenic diabetes insipidus, hypOthyroidism, pregnancy (ebstein anomaly)
29. anhedonia = inability to feel pleasure
30. persistent depressive disorder = dysthymia
    1. MDD at least 2 years in adults
    2. at least 2 of SIGECAPS (except it can be either extreme of appetite and sleep)
    3. symptom free <2 months
    4. must never have been manic or hypomanic
    5. more common in women
31. cyclothymic disorder = at least 2 years = not quite bipolar = doesn't quite meet criteria for a hypomanic episodes or meet criteria for major depressive episode
    1. symptom free <2 months
    2. cant have history of major depressive episode or manic episode
    3. associated with borderline personality disorder
    4. equal in males and females
32. premenstrual dysphoric disorder = PMS
    1. to diagnose, keep MENSTRUAL DIARY
    2. first line tx = SSRI; second line tx = another SSRI
    3. oral contraceptives can also tx if not wanting kids

ANXIETY, OCD, ETC.

1. first line for anxiety = SSRI or SNRI
2. acute panic attack tx = benzo
3. public speaking phobia tx = beta blocker; CI = ASTHMA, if asthma then give = BENZO
4. panic disorder = suddenly out of the blue, unexpected panic attacks with worry for >1 month for getting another attack
    1. smoking, childhood abuse are associated risk factors
    2. higher in women
    3. happens in 20s
    4. panic disorder rx = SSRI , 2nd line = TCA, can use with benzo prn as a bridging med til SSRI works
    5. benzos can also be used for acute panic attack episodes
    6. vs PHEOCHROMOCYTOMA which has HEADACHES + HTN
    7. must rule out life threateners such as MI, thyroid storm, and PE for patients with panic attack sx
    8. screen pts with panic attacks for suicide because increased risk
5. agoraphobia = fear in public especially where escape or help is hard to find for 6 months+
    1. rx = CBT + SSRI
    2. strong genetic factor
    3. usually occurs after traumatic event
    4. causes social or occupational dysfxn
6. social anxiety disorder = social phobia = PUBLIC = fear of embarrassment and getting made fun of in <u>public</u> >6 months
    1. common triggers: public restaurants, public speaking, public restrooms
    2. vs avoidant personality disorder = fear of inadequacy, afraid of rejection = wants to make friends but doesn't

know how

7. first line rx for specific phobia or social anxiety disorder = CBT (SSRI if debilitating)
8. selective mutism = failure to speak in select social situations with sx >1 month
    1. rx = CBT + SSRI
9. separation anxiety disorder = starts 12-18 months
    1. fear from separation from attachment figures
    2. reluctant to leave home or go to school or work
    3. complains of physical sx so they can stay home
    4. qualified if >1 month in kids and teens and >6 months in adults
    5. rx = CBT + SSRI
10. buspirone = 5ht partial agonist used for generalized anxiety disorder
11. generalized anxiety disorder = excessive worrying about everything, restless, muscle tension, insomnia
    1. difficult to control worry
    2. excessive worry >6 months
    3. higher in women
    4. average age is 30 yo
    5. poor prognosis for full recovery
    6. rx = CBT + SSRI
12. OCD dsm 5 = associated with tourettes, high comorbidity with other anxiety disorders
    1. rx = EXPOSURE RESPONSE CONTROL + SSRI
13. ego dystonic = distressed
14. ego syntonic = not distressed
15. body dymorphic disorder = cannot be secondary to eating disorder, preoccupied with body parts and think it is flawed, spend lots of time trying to fix it eg michael jackson, associated with childhood abuse + first degree relatives with OCD, starts

at age 15, high rate of suicide attempts
    1. rx = SSRI + CBT
16. hoarding disorder = clinically significant distress impaired social or occupational functioning, usually older ppl, 50% of people with hoarding also have a relative who hoards
    1. rx = specialized CBT
17. trichotillomania = repeated attempts to decrease or stop hair pulling
    1. rx = SSRI + CBT
18. excoriation/skin picking disorder = majority are women, rx = CBT
19. PTSD = life threatening trauma at anytime in past, sx last 1+ month
    1. life threatening event
    2. nightmares
    3. hyper vigilant/on edge
    4. negative mood
    5. rx = SSRI + CBT
    6. rx nightmare = prazosin
20. Acute Stress Disorder = trauma must have been recent/less than 1 month ago, symptoms <1 month
21. acute stress disorder -> PTSD if greater than 1 month
22. adjustment disorder = stressful life event like divorce, break up, loss of job, not life threatening tho
    1. doesn't quite meet depression criteria
    2. some life event must have happened less than 3 months ago
    3. must cause social/occupational dysfxn
    4. sx resolve within 6 months after stressor has terminated
    5. rx = SUPPORTIVE psychotherapy
    6. if u are stuck picking between grief vs adjustment disorder = if someone recently died, pick grief

23. CBT first line = hoarding, specific phobia, social phobia, hoarding, OCD = think of behavioral things = drugs are less likely to treat

PERSONALITY DISORDERS

1. personality disorders must cause impairment in social or occupational functioning
2. prevalence of all personality disorders = 6%
3. paranoid personality = suspicious, distrust, jealous of others, quick to counterattack, holds grudges, mostly men
    1. uses projection mechanism = accusing another person of the thoughts, feelings, motives that you yourself have
4. schizoid = mostly men, prefer to be alone (avoidant does not want to be alone), rx = day program or drop in centers (schizoids avoid)
5. antisocial = 18 yo+ = main finding is that they commit crimes and don't care about laws or rules = (fighting, burning, stealing, cruelty) more prevalent in males, low socioeconomic rx = none
    1. conduct disorder = <18 yo, tx = behavior modification
    2. oppositional defiant = doesn't commit crimes tho, think of this as more rebellious attitude
    3. conduct disorder -> antisocial if 18 yo+
6. borderline personality disorder = 3x more in women, rapid changes in mood unlike bipolar, uses extremes of language, impulsive, suicidal behavior, uses splitting rx = DBT aka dialectical behavior therapy, associated with cyclothymia (MUST KNOW)
7. histrionic = attention seeking, wears revealing clothes, women more common, defense mechanism is regression
8. narcissistic = wants status and recognition, feels entitled to get better treatment than others = get depressed midlife since they value youth and power
9. OCPD = wants to get the task done perfectly, egosyntonic tho vs OCD which is egodystonic
10. avoidant personality disorder = desires friendship but extremely

shy and doesn't want rejection, males = females, feels inferior to others

11. social anxiety disorder = fear of embarrassment in public
12. avoidant personality disorder = overall fear in general in any situation can be in public can be anywhere, also lifelong
13. dependent personality = need to be taken care of, submissive, clingy, can't stand being alone, allows others to make decisions for them, women more common, defense mechanism = regression
14. specific phobia = inanimate object phobia rx = systemic desensitization therapy

SUBSTANCE ABUSE AND ADDICTION

1. substance induced mood symptoms improve with abstinence where as primary does not
2. alcohol lasts in urine for a few hours, opioids amphetamines cocaine pcp lasts less than 1 week, marijuana diazepam lasts up to 1 month
3. PCP = elevated CPK (creatine phosphokinase) + NYSTAGMUS + VIOLENT
4. alcohol = increased GABA DA and 5HT, inhibits glutamate receptors and voltage calcium channels
    1. BAL >100 shows signs of intoxication, ataxia and poor balance
    2. at BAL of 400+ = potentially fatal
    3. anion gap metabolic acidosis
    4. alcohol withdrawal can kill u; 2 types of withdrawal that can be fatal = alcohol and benzodiazepine
    5. seizures start around 12-24 hours
    6. DTs starts at around 2-4 days after last drink
    7. tx of alcohol withdrawal = lorazepam
    8. banana bag for alcoholic nutritional deficiencies = thiamine, folate, multivitamin
    9. withdrawal signs and symptoms of etoh = clinical institute withdrawal assessment scale (CIWA)
    10. alcoholic with previous withdraw with seizure must be admitted to hospital if they want to detox to watch closely
    11. AUDIT C = screening for alcohol use disorder
    12. alcohol use disorder first line rx = naltrexone or acamprosate
    13. acamprosate = nmda blocker, modulates glu transmission, used for relapse prevention,

ADVANTAGE IS CAN BE USED IN LIVER
DISEASE, CI IN RENAL DISEASE

14. disulfiram = blocks acetaldehyde dehydrogenase = build up of acetaldehyde which produces nausea; should only be given to patients who are super motivated, rarely the first option

15. AST to ALT ratio >2 and elevated GGT = alcohol use

5. cocaine = increased DA, EPI, NE
    1. fever tx = ice bath
    2. od first line tx = benzo
    3. agitation tx = haloperidol
    4. withdrawal of cocaine is not life threatening resolves in 72 hrs
    5. can die due to arrhythmias, mi, or seizure or resp depression
    6. can present like psychosis but they key features are tachycardia, dilated pupils, elevated blood pressure, diaphoresis, NO NYSTAGMUS vs (PCP which has nystagmus)

6. amphetamine = increased NE DA
    1. adderall, crystal meth, MDMA
    2. MDMA = increased DA, NE, 5ht
    3. intox sx = similar to cocaine
    4. tx = rehydrate, correct electrolytes

7. PCP = NMDA blocker and increase DA
    1. rotary nystagmus is very specific sign
    2. VIOLENT, psychotic
    3. rx = benzo or haloperidol

8. dextroamphetamine safer than methylphenidate because doesnt have LEUKOPENIA OR ANEMIA

9. benzos and barbs synergistic with etoh and opioids = can precipitate overdose

10. rx for benzo or barb overdose (OD) = activated charcoal to prevent absorption
    1. or barbs = sodium bicarb to promote renal excretion
    2. or benzo = flumazenil
    3. flumazenil can cause seizures if person is dependent on them, best use for acute OD in first time users
    4. withdrawal can be LIFE THREATENING (seizures)
    5. withdrawal rx = benzo taper
11. withdrawals from downers (benzo, barbs, etoh) can be LIFE THREATENING but uppers (cocaine, pcp, amphetamines) are not life threatening
12. classic triad of opioid OD = resp depression, altered mental status, miosis
13. meperidine = ONLY OPIOID THAT DOES NOT HAVE MIOSIS, DILATES INSTEAD
14. methadone = GOLD STANDARD FOR PREGNANT OPIOID ADDICT = REDUCES MORTALITY RATE = CAUSES LONG QT
15. eating lots of poppy seeds bagels can cause opioid drug screen false positive
16. suboxone = ORAL = buprenorphine + naloxone; naloxone is not active PO, but active IV; if melted and administered IV, will be very unpleasant for user = discourages IV abuse
17. opioid withdrawal tx = supportive = clonidine, nsaids
    1. severe sx tx = buprenorphine or methadone
    2. opioid withdrawal sx = diarrhea, myalgia, rhinorrhea, piloerection
    3. exception for downer, OPIOID WITHDRAWAL NOT LIFE THREATENING
18. hallucinogen intoxication tx = BENZO
19. inhalants like glue = CNS depressant can be fatal due to resp depression or arrhythmias

1. signs = GLUE SNIFFERS RASH = PERIORAL DERMATITIS, very acute onset and resolution of psychotic symptoms
20. caffeine = adenosine antagonist, can cause arrhythmias, seizures at high doses rx = supportive
    1. withdrawal = headache, muscle pain, resolves in 1 week
21. nicotine addiction tx =
    1. varenicline = partial nicotinic acetylcholine receptor agonist, reduces reward; side effect = may increase suicidality
    2. bupropion = NDRI, reduces craving; contraindicated in hx of seizures, alcoholics, bulimia/anorexia because bupropion lowers seizure threshold (MUST KNOW)
22. gambling disorder tx = gamblers anonymous + CBT
23. substance use withdrawal can look like depression especially cocaine and amphetamines
    1. as a principle: think opposite of what the drug does = crash/withdrawal
    2. cocaine withdrawal = depression, sleeps lots, eats lots
    3. amphetamine withdrawal = depression, can't sleep, eat lots

NEUROCOGNITIVE DISORDERS

1. risk factors for delirium = elderly on lots of meds
2. meds that cause delirium = benzos, TCA, anticholinergics
3. delirium EEG = diffuse background slowing
4. delirium tremens EEG = fast activity
5. child delirium cause = febrile illness or meds
6. delirium + dilated pupils + tachycardia = do urine toxicology screen for drugs
7. delirium screening test = confusion assessment method (CAM)
8. mild neurocognitive disorder (mild NCD) = able to maintain independence
9. major neurocognitive disorder (major NCD) = needs help with IADL and ADL
10. dementia is a type of NCD that is IRREVERSIBLE
11. reversible NCDs examples are = b12 deficiency, thyroid problem, NPH
12. apathetic thyrotoxicosis = paradoxical signs of thyrotoxicosis in the elderly aka lethargic
13. alzheimers = decrease memory learning and language = key in vignette is indolent worsening, getting LOST on the way home
    1. extraneuronal beta amyloid
    2. intraneuronal tau fibrillary tangles
    3. apolipoprotein E4 = EARLY dementia
    4. clinical dx
14. antipsychotics = INCREASE MORTALITY CHANCES IN PATIENTS WITH DEMENTIA (BLACK BOX)
15. vascular dementia = STEPWISE DECLINE, has an episode, gets worse, stays like that for a while, gets another hit, then gets worse again like a staircase, look for atherosclerotic, HTN risk factors in patient
16. parkinson's/lewy body dementia adjunct tx

1. dementia tx = cholinesterase inhibitors = donepezil, galantamine, rivastigmine
2. hallucinations tx = quetiapine or clozapine = use short term only b/c incr mortality
3. parkinsonism tx = levodopa carbidopa
4. lewy bodies found in both of them = made of alpha synuclein

17. Frontotemporal dementia rx = PERSONALITY CHANGES, inappropriate behavior, tx = SSRI or trazodone
18. huntington's disease = autosomal dominant, all vignettes will mention a parent who had it and died at age 40, cognitive decline, chorea/motor decline
    1. rx = tetrabenazine or atypical antipsychotics
19. prion disease CJD = startle myoclonus + rapid progression within months
    1. pathology = spongiform cortex
    2. EEG = triphasic/periodic sharp wave complexes
    3. CSF 1433 proteins
20. NPH = enlarged ventricles, but normal pressure on LP, wacky wobbly wet = dementia, ataxia, urinary incontinence
    1. initial tx = lumbar puncture to temporarily lower pressure, definitive tx= ventriculoperitoneal shunt
21. Absence seizures = child who zones out WITHOUT postictal period, EEG = 3 hz spike
    1. vs. complex partial = child who zones out/smacks lips WITH postictal period

GERIATRICS

1. normal aging = decreased brain weight, increased fat, loss of hearing, benign forgetfulness
2. major depression after stroke or MI 3-4x more likely to die
3. pseudodementia = forgetfulness secondary to MDD
    1. when asked about things they will say they don't know but ppl with real dementia will just make stuff up
    2. no sundowning
    3. onset more acute
    4. improves with antidepressants
4. sundowning = increased confusion at night seen in dementia
5. METHYLPHENIDATE = CAUSES INSOMNIA AND ARRHYTHMIAS + ELEVATED BP + LEUKOPENIA + ANEMIA
6. ABNORMAL GRIEF = WORTHLESS, SUICIDAL IDEATION, PERSISTENT PAST 6 MONTHS
7. old ppl have lower levels of alcohol dehydrogenase, lower water in body which causes higher BAL
8. old ppl have weaker kidneys and livers which causes drugs to build up faster
9. drinking can exacerbate gout, diabetes, hypertension
10. metronidazole, sulfonamides, sulfonylurea = disulfiram like reaction n/v
11. most common psychiatric disorder in elderly = MDD
12. white elderly males with substance abuse have highest rate of completed suicide
13. if u must use antipsychotics aka aggression, hallucination, psychosis in old ppl, which is dangerous = OLDMANZAPINE OR QUIETIPAINE = because OLD MAN wants it QUIET
14. Restless leg syndrome = feeling of restlessness in legs, uncomfortable feeling almost like u have to get up and move,

can be distressing, tx = dopamine agonist = ropinirole, pramipexole = associated with iron deficiency anemia, can be confusing with akathisia but the key is that in restless leg syndrome there is no history of taking antipsychotics

15. Elderly changes in sleep patterns:
    1. decreased REM = less dreams
    2. increase stage 1 and 2, decreased stage 3 and 4 = light sleepers
    3. goes to sleep earlier, wakes up earlier = early birds
16. Bruxism = teeth grinding = N2 stage (MUST KNOW)
17. Night terrors = N3 stage (MUST KNOW)
18. elderly abuse prime suspect = CAREGIVER
19. don't use these drugs in elderly = antipsychotic (mortality, use short term only), anticholinergic, antihistamines, benzos (paradoxical agitation)
20. SAFEST SLEEPY PILL IN ELDERLY = TRAZODONE
    1. trazodone side effect = ORTHOSTATIC HYPOTENSION, priapism

PEDIATRIC PSYCHIATRY

1. KABC = kaufman assessment battery for children = intelligence test between 2-12 yo
2. WISCR = wechsler intelligence scale for children = IQ test 6-16 yo
3. Fragile X = most common inherited form of intellectual disability
4. down syndrome = most common chromosomal disorder (this does not qualify as inherited because it is a sporadic event)
5. language disorder = expressive/receptive impairment = low vocab, doesn't understand language
6. speech sound disorder = cannot articulate well = lisp
7. fluency disorder = stuttering
8. ADHD = at least 6 months of symptoms, onset SX MUST BE PRESENT BEFORE AGE 12 aka if you truly have ADHD, you would have had it since you were a kid
9. fragile x = most common single gene cause of ASD (autism)
10. tourettes = COMBO OF multiple motor tics AND 1 vocal tic for 1 YEAR+ (does not have to occur together), MUST HAVE STARTED BEFORE AGE 18
    1. motor tic = blinking, shrugging
    2. vocal tic = coprolalia, echolalia
    3. first line tx = habit reversal therapy
    4. second line tx = atypical antipsychotics or guanfacine (alpha 2 agonist)
11. persistent motor or vocal tic disorder = chronic tics, NEVER BOTH
12. provisional tic disorder = less than 1 yr of sx
13. oppositional defiant disorder rx = BEHAVIOR MODIFICATION
    1. does not get aggressive or physical vs conduct disorder

which does and does criminal acts

14. conduct disorder = breaks laws, gets into fights, steals stuff
    1. RX = BEHAVIOR MODIFICATION
    2. female conduct disorder manifestations = prostitution, lying, running away, substance abuse
15. PRIMARY elimination disorder = never potty trained
16. SECONDARY elimination disorder = was potty trained, but then became untrained
17. enuresis = bedwetting/untrained urination
    1. must be >5 yo; U R I N E = 5 letters
    2. must have been a problem for 3 months straight
    3. first line tx = URINE ALARM, second line tx = DESMOPRESSIN third line tx = IMIPRAMINE (TCA)
    4. females more likely for day peeing (diurnal enuresis)
    5. males more likely for night peeing (nocturnal enuresis)
18. encopresis = untrained pooping
    1. must be >4 yo = P O O P = 4 letters
    2. must have been a problem for 3 months straight
19. majority of enuresis cases will resolve on their own with time
20. alcohol is most common drug of abuse in teens
21. doctors are "mandated reporters" = legally required to report all causes of suspected child abuse
22. ADHD has to have started before 12
23. tourettes has to have started before age 18
24. SPIRAL BONE FRACTURE = suspected abuse

DISSOCIATIVE DISORDERS

1. dissociative amnesia = major life stressor that made the person forget their identity = usually will be found lost not knowing who are where they are
    1. tx = supportive, CBT, hypnosis
    2. increased risk for suicide when memories come back
    3. often these pts are also suffering from MDD
2. depersonalization/derealization = also associated with major life stressor but u feel like u are having out of body experiences or watching yourself from 3rd person
    1. tx = CBT, hypnosis, supportive
3. dissociative identity disorder = multiple personality disorder = usually in victims of physical/sexual abuse, neglect, PTSD, 70% will try to kill themselves, worst prognosis of all dissociative disorders
    1. Tx = psychotherapy
    2. Tx pharm = combination = SSRI for depression and PTSD, prazosin for nightmares, and naltrexone for self mutilation

SOMATIC SYMPTOM, FACTITIOUS, AND OTHER DISORDERS

1. somatic symptom disorder = 6 months+ of pain/sx, complaints of multiple organ system problems, pain, nervous system, diarrhea etc WITHOUT a DX aka u cannot find an explanation
    1. tx = REGULAR VISITS TO FAMILY DOC (MUST KNOW)
    2. don't confuse with generalized anxiety disorder which can include somatic symptoms but the patient will often be stressed out about everything in their life social, work, family, and including their own body - whereas somatic symptom disorder is preoccupied about the body only
2. conversion disorder tx = life stressor -> neurologic deficit that is unexplained medically
    1. tx = EDUCATION ABOUT ILLNESS, CAN DO CBT IF EDUCATION DOESN'T WORK
3. illness anxiety disorder = 6 MONTHS+ of worry about getting or having an illness, no complaints of pain or sx tho, tx = regular visits to family doc
4. factitious disorder/munchausen = pretending to be ill, motive is for attention/care from others
5. malingering = faking illness, motive is for personal gain like not wanting to go back to prison, taking time off work, lawsuit etc
6. intermittent explosive disorder = intermittent explosive rages of anger
    1. tx = CBT + SSRI
    2. low serotonin in CSF
7. kleptomania = stealing but the person doesn't really need it for anything, just feels good to steal

1. rx = CBT + SSRI (CBT = desensitization, aversion conditioning)
2. strong association with bulimia nervosa (2/3 of patients have bulimia)

8. pyromania = urge to burn things, tx = CBT + SSRI

EATING DISORDERS

1. Anorexic medical complications (Everything goes low):
    1. unhealthy caloric deficit
    2. low BMI is KEY vs bulimia = NORMAL BMI (MUST KNOW)
    3. cardiac = bradycardia, anemia, leukopenia
    4. hypokalemia, low electrolytes
2. anorexia 2 types:
    1. restricting type = does not vomit
    2. binge purge type = vomits after eating just a little bit
3. anorexia admit to hospital if: unstable vitals, electrolyte disturbances
4. anorexia common in activities that have social pressure to look good
5. refeeding syndrome = sudden drop in phosphorous = first meal after a long period of starvation (Excess use of hexokinase during glycolysis), mg, ca; sx = arrhythmia, resp failure, delirium, seizures (MUST KNOW)
6. anorexia predisposed to osteoporosis and stress fractures amenorrhea
7. anorexia tx = FOOD + CBT
8. Bulimia = binge and purge at least once a week for 3 MONTHS+ = NORMAL BMI
    1. russell's sign = callouses/abrasions on back of hand
9. anorexia associated with OCD, Bulimia associated with BPD
10. anorexics usually have HIGH CORTISOL STRESS
11. anorexia/bulimia -> hypokalemia -> arrhythmia
12. anorexia worse prognosis than bulimia
13. BULIMIA FIRST LINE TX = FLUOXETINE + CBT
14. BUPROPION CI = EATING DISORDER BECAUSE SEIZURE THRESHOLD LOWERED

15. binge eating disorder = 3+ MONTHS of excessive eating habits, BMI = 30+
    1. eating too much till it hurts even when u aren't hungry and embarrassed about it
    2. eats in private
    3. first line tx = stimulants (decreases appetite) + CBT
16. obesity weight loss first line tx = lifestyle modification, second line tx = orlistat (pancreatic lipase inhibitor)

SLEEPING DISORDERS

1. REM -> transient htn, tachycardia, tachypnea (INCREASE ALL VITALS, its like ur waking/revving up)
2. first line tx insomnia = good sleep hygiene
3. Z drugs = zolpidem, zaleplon, zopiclone; main side effect = orthostatic hypotension
    1. orthostatic hypotension side effect drugs = maoi, trazodone, z drugs
4. zolpidem CI in elderly = causes falls, cognitive impairment
5. depression + insomnia tx = trazodone, mirtazapine
6. hypersomnolence disorder = excessive sleep but still tired after, 3+ months
    1. ddx = mono, HIV, guillain barre
    2. tx = modafinil or methylphenidate + napping schedules
7. tx for obstructive sleep apnea = CPAP (continuous airway positive pressure), weight loss, exercise, surgery
8. cheyne stokes breathing = periodic crescendo decrescendo tidal volume caused by HF, stroke, renal failure, opiates
    1. rx = treat underlying condition, CPAP, supplement o2
9. narcolepsy = diminished hypocretin/orexin in CSF = hormone that keeps you awake, goes into REM sleep very quickly on polysomnography
    1. will have problems staying awake, falls asleep suddenly + CATAPLEXY
    2. cataplexy = sudden loss of muscle tone by strong emotion while staying conscious = KEY FEATURE
    3. loss of hypothalamic neurons that produce hypocretin
    4. first line tx = MODAFINIL
10. severe shift work disorder of sleep tx = modafinil
11. delayed/advanced sleep disorder = early bird or night owl = timed bright light therapy

12. sleepwalking risk factor = sleep deprivation, self resolves, but in severe cases tx = LOW DOSE BENZO (clonazepam)
13. sleep terror = appears to have violent nightmares but does not remember dream, because during stage N3 not REM, tx = self limited, benign, just reassure
14. nightmare disorder = can easily remember all the details of the nightmare, a/w PTSD
    1. tx = desensitization/imagery rehearsal therapy = modifying the outcome of the recurrent nightmare
    2. PTSD nightmares tx = prazosin
    3. happens during REM sleep
15. REM sleep behavior disorder = dream acting, sleep talking, walking, running, can be dangerous for family members and patient
    1. associated with underlying NCD
    2. tx = clonazepam or melatonin or discontinue psych meds
16. restless leg syndrome tx = dopamine agonist = ropinirole or pramipexole
    1. can be caused by meds or iron deficiency

SEXUAL DISORDERS

1. male hypoactive sexual desire disorder = deficiency of sexual thoughts, desires, fantasies for 6+ months
    1. tx = testosterone
2. female sexual interest/arousal disorder = deficiency in interest, thoughts, sensations for 6+ months
    1. tx = vaginal estrogen or systemic testosterone
3. erectile disorder = 6+ months
    1. must rule out psychological causes via nocturnal erections; if nocturnal erections = psychological ED, but if they don't get them most likely this is a physiological ED
    2. if caused by atherosclerosis = PDE5 inhibitor = sildenafil oral
4. premature ejaculation = ejaculation in less than 1 minute for 6+months
    1. rx = SSRI/TCA
    2. tx = squeeze the glans before ejaculation, stopping touching before ejaculation
5. genitopelvic pain/penetration disorder = vaginismus = dyspareunia for 6+months
    1. key feature is pain upon superficial entry to the vagina
    2. gradual desensitization muscle relaxation -> massage -> intercourse
6. vulvodynia = allodynia of the vulva very sensitive to pain/touch; first line tx = physiotherapy
7. gender dysphoria = transsexual/transgender
    1. begins around age 3 when gender identity is established
    2. wants to be the opposite gender
    3. rx for young ppl = therapy and family involvement
    4. surgical sex change = only after living in 1 year of

gender role and 1 year of hormone therapy
8. pedophilic disorder = must be at least 16 yo to 11 yo age gap
9. sadist = like others to suffer = dominatrix
10. masochist = likes self suffering

PSYCHOTHERAPIES

1. sublimation = taking something destructive and making it constructive that is an advantage/benefit for u = mature defense mechanism
2. mature defense mechanisms = SASH = sublimation, altruism, suppression, humor
3. operant conditioning = reward/punishment system
4. systematic desensitization = specific phobia = relaxation techniques level 1 -> increasing levels of phobia stimuli
5. negative reinforcement = removing painful stimulus
6. aversion therapy = positive punishment, adding something unpleasant

PHARMACOLOGY

1. serotonin syndrome can cause rhabdomyolysis -> renal failure
2. serotonin syndrome has myoclonus/tremors vs nms has rigidity and elevated cpk
    1. also key hack is to look at what drug they took in the vignette, if they took an SSRI = probably serotonin syndrome, if they took an antipsychotic, probably neuroleptic malignant syndrome
3. cough syrup (dextromethorphan) can precipitate serotonin syndrome when mixed with SSRI/MAOI
4. fluoxetine = prozac = safe in pregnancy and kids
5. paroxetine = teratogenic = pulmonary htn in fetus; quickest half life can precipitate withdrawal
6. VENLAFAXINE tx = fibromyalgia, NEUROPATHIC PAIN
7. snri think ssri side effects + hypertension
8. duloxetine rx = fibromyalgia, neuropathic pain
    1. se = hepatotoxic
9. bupropion = used for smoking quitting and depression, no sexual side effects, no weight gain, lowers seizure threshold
    1. contraindicated in = eating disorder, seizure disorder, ppl taking MAOI
10. traZZZoBone tx = MDD with insomnia (SSRI)
    1. main se = sleepy, orthostatic hypotension, priapism
11. mirtaZZZapine rx = MDD with insomnia and low appetite
    1. helps u ZZZ and helps u eat to gain weight
    2. safe in elderly
12. Antimuscarinic drugs can make acute angle glaucoma worse via mydriasis = plugs up trabecular meshwork = decreased aqueous humor drainage
13. signs of lithium overdose = ataxia, dysarthria, delirium; hx of lithium use

14. MAOI use = prevents breakdown of tyramine; cheese, smoked meats -> tyrosine -> tyramine -> NE -> HTN crisis
15. MOST COMMON SIDE EFFECT OF MAOI = ORTHOSTATIC HYPOTENSION
16. serotonin syndrome rx = discontinue meds, supportive, benzos or cyproheptadine
17. insomnia + depression tx = mirtazapine, trazodone
18. neuropathic pain drugs = TCA or SNRI
19. chronic pain/fibromyalgia = SNRI, TCA
20. atypical antipsychotics are very dangerous in elderly and can cause them to die and get strokes (use with caution if elderly person is acting psychotic)
21. haloperidol DECANOATE = LONG ACTING FORM
22. akathisia rx = beta blocker, benzo
23. restless leg syndrome rx = dopamine agonist
24. high potency typical antipsychotics haloperidol IM are first line for acute agitation/psychosis
25. NMS sx = FALTERED = fever, autonomic instability, leukocytosis, tremor, elevated cpk, rigidity, excess sweating, delirium
26. NMS rx = discontinue, supportive -> bromocriptine, dantrolene, amantadine
27. washout period for fluoxetine = 5-6 weeks cuz its half life is the longest of SSRI, the rest only needs 2 week washout = important to know when starting another drug
28. clozapine se = myocarditis, agranulocytosis, seizures = LEAST RISK FOR TARDIVE
29. risperidone main SE = prolactinemia, orthostatic hypotension
30. ziprasidone SE = long QT
31. atypical antipsychotic main SE = metabolic, HAM block (histamine, alpha, muscarinic), liver damage, long QT
32. only mood stabilizer to decrease suicide = lithium (MUST

KNOW)

33. only antipsychotic to decrease suicide = clozapine (MUST KNOW)
34. therapeutic range of lithium = 0.6-1.2 (same as creatinine) toxic = 1.5+
35. things that elevated Li+ levels = nsaids, aspirin, thiazides, dehydration = kidney drugs
36. rapid cycling bipolar rx = mood stabilizer = valproate or carbamazepine
37. valproate = blocks Na channels and increase GABA = CAUSES NTD
38. NTD neural tube defect drugs = carbamazepine and valproate
39. VALPROATE MAIN SE = ALOPECIA, HEPATOTOXIC, PANCREATITIS, NTD, THROMBOCYTOPENIA = check CBC and LFTs
40. buspirone = partial 5ht agonist
41. methylphenidate can cause leukopenia, anemia
42. atomoxetine = NRI = non addicting for ADHD tx, not first line, but less efficacy than methylphenidate/dextroamphetamine
43. drug classes that cause sedation, confusion = anticholinergics, antihistamines, benzos
44. drug that causes depression = corticosteroids
45. most efficacy rx for MDD, MANIA, CATATONIA = ECT
    1. use if pt cannot tolerate or if meds dont work
46. quitting smoking tx = bupropion, varenicline
47. quitting drinking tx = acamprosate, naltrexone
48. ibs tx = ssri
49. chronic pain/neuropathic rx = tca/snri
50. fibromyalgia rx = snri, tca
51. pms rx = ssri
52. hiccups tx = chlorpromazine

53. patient taking clozapine and develops agranulocytosis, next step = stop clozapine (MUST KNOW)
54. schizoaffective = antipsychotic + MOOD STABILIZER
55. valproate also check CBC and LFT
56. partial agonists
    1. aripiprazole = partial dopamine antagonist = antipsychotic
    2. buprenorphine = partial opioid agonist = opioid addiction
    3. buspirone = partial serotonin agonist = generalized anxiety disorder
    4. varenicline = partial nicotinic acetylcholine receptor agonist = quit smoking
57. clozapine = least likely to cause EPS/tardive dyskinesia, most potent antipsychotic that can minimize suicide risk the best, however can cause agranulocytosis; if patient gets signs of infection = check CBC and discontinue clozapine
58. ATYPICAL SIDE EFFECT KEY DIFFERENCES U NEED TO KNOW:
    1. clozapine = famous for LEAST CHANCE OF tardive dyskinesia
    2. quetiapine = famous for LEAST movement disorder
    3. olanzapine = famous for weight gain and diabetes
    4. risperidone = famous for movement disorders, prolactinemia, hypotension
    5. ziprasidone = famous for LONG QT
59. first gen high potency antipsychotic SE = EPS = fluphenazine + haloperidol;
    1. first gen low potency SE = HAM block = chlorpromazine, thioridazine
    2. second gen SE = metabolic syndrome = clozapine, quetiapine, risperidone, olanzapine, aripiprazole

60. bipolar mood stabilizers = VLC = valproate, lithium, carbamazepine
61. Alzheimer drugs = acetylcholinesterase inhibitors = Grandma Doesn't Remember MeMan= galantamine, rivastigmine, donepezil, memantine

MISCELLANEOUS

1. dealbreakers for confidentiality = subpoena, child abuse, suicidal, dangerous to self/others
2. doesn't need consent = unconscious lifesaving emergency (implied consent), prevention of suicide/homicide (involuntary hospitalization)
3. emancipated minors = self supporting, married, military, pregnant or has kids = can give their own consent and make own medical decisions
4. involuntary psych hold = harmful to self, others, can't take care of self
5. 4 Rs of informed consent:
    1. reason for tx
    2. risk vs benefits
    3. reasonable alternatives
    4. refused tx consequences
6. most important risk factor in assessing a pt risk of violence = history of violence
7. must respect patients wishes of autonomy if it's not an immediately life threatening emergency but may kill them, u still have to respect their decision
8. reference = tv character sending patient messages
9. insight = awareness/understanding of patient's own problem, if patient has poor insight about own problem u have to be careful with your approach and not shock them
10. judgment = understanding outcome of patient's own actions
11. alcoholic hallucinosis = 6-12 hours in, during or right after heavy drinking, hearing sounds, aware that not real, vital signs normal, no clouding of sensorium
12. DTs = 2-4 days in, poor vitals, clouding of sensorium rx = benzos

13. prior history of violence is most important predictor of future violence; for most other things as well
14. IQ = mean of 100 with standard deviation of 15
15. Intellectual disability = IQ less than 70 aka 2 standard deviations below
16. Adjustment disorder is not quite depression with social occupational dysfunction with an event that happened less than 3 months ago
    1. adjustment disorder vs bereavement/grief = adjustment disorder has social occupational dysfunctioning but grief does not
    2. grief vs depression = grief comes in waves, depression is constant, depression associated with WORTHLESSNESS
17. dx of sleep apnea = sleep studies aka polysomnography
18. depression neurotransmitters all down vs anxiety all down but NE up
    1. NE, 5ht, DA all down in depression
19. schizophrenia neurotransmitters all up
20. parkinson has low DA but high ACH
21. BEST WAY TO CHECK OVERDOSE OF TCA IS EKG FOR LONG QT USED AS INDICATION FOR SODIUM BICARB THERAPY
22. benzo vs alcohol intoxication = alcohol has nystagmus benzos do not
23. first line for smoking cessation: nicotine patch/gum -> varenicline -> bupropion
24. CONTRAINDICATION TO PUBLIC SPEAKING BETA BLOCKER = ASTHMA, SO INSTEAD U GIVE LORAZEPAM
25. panic disorder vs pheochromocytoma = HYPERTENSION in Pheochromocytoma

26. DX OF EPILEPSY = EEG
27. Elevated CPK = seen in NMS or PCP intoxication
28. Prozac = fluoxetine is most safe for pregnant
29. acute mania with agitation rx = antipsychotic b/c quicker onset, lithium takes too long
30. bupropion doesnt make u gain weight, does not have sexual side effects but lowers seizure threshold
31. Schizophrenia prevalence is ~1% usa
32. Depression prevalence is ~10% usa
33. Death is permanent around 7 yo

About the Author:

Steven Vuu aka Dr. High Yield, is a general surgery resident at the University of Central Florida College of Medicine. He was born and raised in Vancouver, BC, Canada. He completed his medical degree at Ross University School of Medicine, finishing in the top 5% of his class, graduating with Summa Cum Laude (Highest Honors). He was a Dean's Honor Roll and Dean's List student in all 4 years of medical school and scored above 250 and 265 on the USMLE Step 1 and 2 CK exams, respectively. His Step 2 CK score was approximately in the 95th

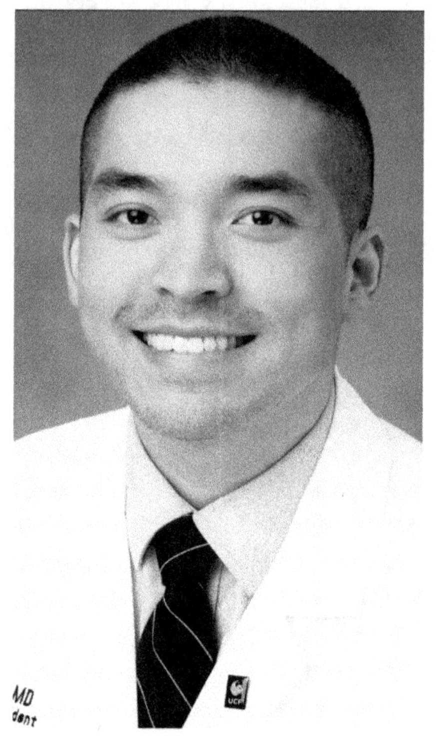

percentile worldwide. He was head TA in medical school, and tutored full classrooms each week in preparation for their exams. There, he learned that he had helped many of his classmates increase their scores. This would eventually set the stage for his future in medical education. Before that, he graduated from The University of British Columbia in Vancouver, BC, Canada with a Bachelor's Degree in Science. During his spare time, he likes to make electronic music, work out, and watch movies.

www.ingramcontent.com/pod-product-compliance
Lightning Source LLC
Chambersburg PA
CBHW051400150726
48000CB00003B/1271